Donald k. Cilley

# THE CORPULENCE (obesity) CAUSE AND SOLUTION

*How to loose weight and overcome obesity*

*First edition*

*This book was professionally typeset on Reedsy*
*Find out more at reedsy.com*

# Contents

# INTRODUCTION: THE CORPULENCE

Corpulence is an intricate illness including an unnecessary measure of muscle versus fat. Corpulence isn't simply a corrective concern. A clinical issue builds the gamble of different sicknesses and medical conditions, for example, coronary illness, diabetes, hypertension and certain diseases.

There are many motivations behind why certain individuals experience issues getting in shape. Normally, weight results from acquired, physiological and ecological variables, joined with diet, actual work and exercise decisions.

Fortunately even unobtrusive weight reduction can improve or forestall the medical conditions related with corpulence. A better eating routine, expanded actual work and conduct changes can assist you with shedding pounds. Doctor prescribed meds and weight reduction strategies are extra choices for treating stoutness.

# CAUSES

In spite of the fact that there are hereditary, social, metabolic and hormonal impacts on body weight, heftiness happens when you take in additional calories than you consume typical day to day exercises and exercise. Your body stores these abundant calories as fat.

In the United States, the vast majority's weight control plans are too high in calories — frequently from cheap food and fatty drinks. Individuals with heftiness could eat more calories prior to feeling full, feel hungry sooner, or eat more because of stress or tension.

Many individuals who live in Western nations currently have occupations that are considerably less truly demanding, so they don't generally consume as many calories at work. Indeed, even day to day exercises utilize less calories, graciousness of comforts like controllers, elevators, internet shopping and drive-through banks.

# SIDE EFFECT

Weight record (BMI) is frequently used to analyze stoutness. To ascertain BMI, duplicate load in pounds by 703, partition by level in inches and afterward partition again by level in inches. Or on the other hand partition weight in kilograms by level in meters squared.

BMI Weight status

Beneath 18.5 Underweight

18.5-24.9 Normal

25.0-29.9 Overweight

30.0 and higher Obesity

Asians with BMI of 23 or higher may have an expanded gamble of medical conditions.

For a great countless people, BMI gives a sensible gauge of muscle to fat ratio. In any case, BMI doesn't straightforwardly gauge muscle versus fat, so certain individuals, like strong competitors, may have a BMI in the weight classification despite the fact that they don't have an overabundance of muscle versus fat.

Many specialists likewise measure an individual's midsection circuit to assist with directing treatment choices. Weight-related medical issues are more normal in men with a midsection perimeter north of 40 inches (102 centimeters) and in ladies with a midriff estimation north of 35 inches (89 centimeters).

When to see a specialist

On the off chance that you're worried about your weight or weight-related medical issues, get some information about corpulence the executives. You and your PCP can assess your well-being chances and talk about your weight reduction choices.

# RISK FACTORS

Corpulence generally results from a blend of causes and contributing elements:

**Family legacy and impacts**

The qualities you acquire from your folks might influence how much muscle versus fat you store, and where that fat is disseminated. Hereditary qualities may likewise assume a part in how productively your body changes over food into energy, how your body manages your hunger and how your body consumes calories during exercise.

Stoutness will in general spat families. That is not a result of the qualities they share. Relatives likewise will generally have comparative eating and action propensities.

**Way of life decisions**

Unfortunate eating regimen. An eating routine that is high in calories, ailing in products of the soil, brimming with cheap food, and loaded down with unhealthy drinks and larger than usual parts adds to weight gain.

**Fluid calories.** Only a respective can drink numerous calories without feeling full, particularly calories from liquor.

Other fatty refreshments, like sugary soda pops, can add to huge weight gain.

**Latency**. In the event that you have a stationary way of life, you can undoubtedly take in additional calories consistently than you consume exercise and routine day to day exercises. Taking a gander at PC, tablet and telephone screens is an inactive action. The quantity of hours spent before a screen is exceptionally connected with weight gain.

Certain illnesses and prescriptions

In certain individuals, stoutness can be followed by a clinical reason, like Prader-Willi disorder, Cushing disorder and different circumstances. Clinical issues, like joint pain, additionally can prompt diminished movement, which might bring about weight gain.

A few drugs can prompt weight gain on the off chance that you don't repay through diet or movement. These drugs incorporate a few antidepressants, hostile to seizure prescriptions, diabetes meds, antipsychotic meds, steroids and beta blockers.

**Social and financial issues**

Social and financial elements are connected to corpulence. Staying away from heftiness is troublesome in the event that you don't have safe regions to walk or exercise. Essentially, you might not have been shown sound approaches to cooking, or you might not approach better food sources.

Furthermore, individuals you invest energy with may impact your weight — you're bound to foster corpulence in the event that you have companions or family members with heftiness.

**Age**

Corpulence can happen at whatever stage in life, even in small kids. However, as you age, hormonal changes and a less dynamic way of life increase your gamble of weight. Also, how much muscle in your body will in general diminish with age. By and large, lower bulk prompts a reduction in digestion. These progressions additionally decrease calorie needs and can make it harder to keep off overabundance weight. In the event that you don't deliberately control what you eat and turn out to be all the more actually dynamic as you age, you'll probably put on weight.

# OTHER FACTORS

**Pregnancy.** Weight gain is normal during pregnancy. A few ladies find this weight challenging to lose after the child is conceived. This weight gain might add to the improvement of heftiness in ladies.

**Stopping smoking.** Stopping smoking is frequently connected with weight gain. What's more, as far as some might be concerned, it can prompt sufficient weight gain to qualify as heftiness. Frequently, this occurs as individuals use food to adapt to smoking withdrawal. Over the long haul, in any case, stopping smoking is as yet a more prominent advantage to your well being than is proceeding to smoke. Your primary care physician can assist you with forestalling weight gain subsequent to stopping smoking.

**Absence of rest.** Not getting sufficient rest or getting an excessive amount of rest can cause changes in chemicals that increment hunger. You may likewise hunger for food sources high in calories and sugars, which can add to weight gain.

**smoke**. Your PCP can assist you with forestalling weight gain subsequent to stopping smoking.

**Stress.** Numerous outer elements that influence state of mind and prosperity might add to heftiness. Individuals frequently look for all the more fatty food while encountering unpleasant circumstances.

**Microbiome.** Your stomach microbes are impacted by what you eat and may add to weight gain or trouble getting thinner.

Regardless of whether you have at least one of these gamble factors, it doesn't imply that you're bound to foster weight. You can balance most gamble factors through diet, active work and exercise, and conduct changes.

**Inconveniences**

Individuals with stoutness are bound to foster various possibly serious medical issues, including:

**Coronary illness and strokes.** Corpulence makes you bound to have hypertension and strange cholesterol levels, which are risk factors for coronary illness and strokes.

**Type 2 diabetes.** Corpulence can influence the manner in which the body utilizes insulin to control glucose levels. This raises the gamble of insulin opposition and diabetes.

**Certain malignant growths.** Weight might expand the gamble of malignant growth of the uterus, cervix, endometrium, ovary, bosom, colon, rectum, throat, liver, gallbladder, pancreas, kidney and prostate.

**Stomach related issues.** Corpulence improves the probability of creating acid reflex, gallbladder infection and liver issues.

**Rest apnea.** Individuals with corpulence are bound to have rest apnea, a possibly serious problem in which breathing over and over stops and starts during rest.

**Osteoarthritis.** Heftiness expands the pressure put on weight-bearing joints, as well as advancing aggravation inside the body. These variables might prompt intricacies like osteoarthritis.

**Extreme COVID-19 side effects.** Stoutness expands the gamble of creating serious side effects assuming you become contaminated with the infection that causes Covid illness 2019 (COVID-19). Individuals who have serious instances of COVID-19 might require therapy in concentrated care units or even mechanical help to relax. serious COVID-19 ailment develops further - Related informationLink between additional pounds, extreme COVID-19 disease develops further

**Personal satisfaction**

Heftiness can decrease general personal satisfaction. You will most likely be unable to do proactive tasks that you used to appreciate. You might keep away from public spots. Individuals with weight might try and experience separation.

Other weight-related issues that might influence your personal satisfaction include:

**Sorrow**

Incapacity

Disgrace and culpability

Social detachment

Lower work accomplishment.

# FINDINGS

To analyze stoutness, your PCP will regularly play out an actual test and suggest a few tests.

**These tests and tests by and large include:**

**Taking your well-being history.** Your PCP might survey your weight history, weight reduction endeavors, actual work and exercise propensities, eating examples and craving control, what different circumstances you've had, meds, feelings of anxiety, and different issues about your well-being. Your PCP may likewise survey your family's well-being history to check whether you might be inclined toward specific circumstances.

**An overall actual test.** This incorporates estimating your level; really taking a look at essential signs, for example, pulse, circulatory strain and temperature; paying attention to your heart and lungs; and inspecting your mid-region.

**Working out your BMI.** Your PCP will check your weight file (BMI). A BMI of 30 or higher is viewed as stoutness. Numbers higher than 30 increment well-being gambles considerably more. Your BMI ought to be checked something like once per year since it can assist with deciding your general well-being dangers and what medicines might be fitting.

**Estimating your midsection periphery.** Fat put away around the midsection, at times called instinctive fat or stomach fat, may additionally expand the gamble of coronary illness and diabetes. Ladies with a midriff estimation (boundary) of more than 35 inches (89 centimeters) and men with a midsection estimation of more than 40 inches (102 centimeters) may have more well-being takes a chance than do individuals with more modest midsection estimations. Like the BMI estimation, midriff boundary ought to be really looked at no less than one time each year.

**Checking for other medical conditions.** Assuming you have known medical conditions, your primary care physician will assess them. Your PCP will likewise check for other conceivable medical conditions, for example, hypertension, elevated cholesterol, underactive thyroid, liver issues and diabetes.

# TREATMENT

The objective of heftiness treatment is to reach and remain at a solid weight. This works on by and large well-being and brings down the gamble of creating complexities connected with corpulence.

You might have to work with a group of well-being experts — including a dietitian, social guide or a heftiness trained professional — to help you comprehend and make changes in your eating and movement propensities.

The underlying treatment objective is generally an unobtrusive weight reduction — 5% to 10% of your complete weight. That truly intends that assuming you weigh 200 pounds (91 kilograms), you'd have to lose something like 10 to 20 pounds (4.5 to 9 kilograms) for your well-being to start to get to the next level. Notwithstanding, the more weight you lose, the more noteworthy the advantages.

All get-healthy plans require changes in your dietary patterns and expanded active work. The treatment strategies that are ideal for you rely upon your heftiness seriousness, your general well-being and your readiness to partake in your weight reduction plan.

**Dietary changes**

Lessening calories and pursuing better eating routines are essential to defeating corpulence. Despite the fact that you might get more fit rapidly right away, consistent weight reduction over the long haul is viewed as the most secure method for shedding pounds and the most effective way to keep it off for all time.

**There is no best weight reduction diet. Pick one that incorporates good food sources that you feel will work for you. Dietary changes to treat corpulence include:**

**Cutting calories.** The way to weight reduction is lessening the number of calories you that take in. The initial step is to audit your average eating and drinking propensities to perceive the number of calories you that typically polish off and where you can scale back. You and your primary care physician can conclude the number of calories you that need to require in every day to get in shape, however a run of the mill sum is 1,200 to 1,500 calories for ladies and 1,500 to 1,800 for men.

**Feeling full on less.** A few food sources — like sweets, confections, fats and handled food varieties — contain a ton of calories for a little part. Interestingly, leafy foods furnish a bigger part size with less calories. By eating bigger bits of food sources that have less calories, you decrease food cravings, take in less calories and rest easier thinking about your dinner, which adds to how fulfilled you feel generally.

**Pursuing better decisions.** To make your general eating regimen better, eat more plant-based food sources, like natural products, vegetables and entire grains. Likewise stress lean wellsprings of protein — like beans, lentils and soy — and lean meats. In the event that you like fish, attempt to incorporate fish two times per week. Limit salt and added sugar. Eat modest quantities of fats, and ensure they come from heart-sound sources, for example, olive, canola and nut oils.

**Limiting specific food varieties.** Certain weight control plans limit how much a specific nutrition type, like high-sugar or full-fat food sources. Ask your primary care physician which diet plans are successful and which may be useful for you. Drinking sugar-improved refreshments is a certain method for polishing off additional calories than you planned. Restricting these beverages or disposing of them through and through is a decent spot to begin cutting calories.

**Dinner substitutions.** These plans recommend supplanting a couple of feasts with their items —, for example, low-calorie shakes or dinner bars — and practice good eating habits snacks and a solid, adjusted third dinner that is low in fat and calories. Temporarily, this sort of diet can assist you with getting thinner. Be that as it may, these eating regimens probably won't show you how to change your general way of life. So you might need to remain on the eating routine if you have any desire to keep your weight off.

**Be careful about convenient solutions.** You might be enticed by trend slims down that commitment quick and simple weight reduction. The truth, in any case, is that there are no enchanted food sources or convenient solutions. Trend diets might help temporarily, yet the drawn out results don't seem, by all accounts, to be any better compared to different eating regimens.

Essentially, you might get thinner on an accident diet, however you're probably going to recapture it when you stop the eating regimen. To get in shape — and keep it off — you should embrace smart dieting propensities that you can keep up with over the long run.

**Exercise and action**

Expanded actual work or exercise is a fundamental piece of corpulence treatment:

**Work out.** Individuals with stoutness need to get no less than 150 minutes per seven day stretch of moderate-power active work to forestall further weight gain or to keep up with the departure of a humble measure of weight. You most likely should step by step build the sum you practice as your perseverance and wellness get to the next level.

**Continue to move.** Despite the fact that customary oxygen consuming activity is the most proficient method for consuming calories and shed overabundance weight, any additional development helps consume calories. Park farther from store doorways and use the stairwell rather than the lift. A pedometer can follow the number of steps you that assume control throughout the span of a day. Many individuals attempt to arrive at 10,000 stages consistently. Bit by bit increment the quantity of advances you take day to day to arrive at that objective.

**Conduct changes**

A change in behavior patterns program can assist you with making way of life changes and get thinner and keep it off. Moves toward take incorporate looking at your ongoing propensities to figure out what elements, stresses or circumstances might have added to your corpulence.

**Advising.** Chatting with a psychological well-being proficient can assist with resolving profound and social issues connected with eating. Treatment can assist you with understanding the reason why you indulge and learn solid ways of adapting to tension. You can likewise figure out how to screen your eating routine and movement, grasp eating triggers, and adapt to food desires. Guiding can be one-on-one or in a gathering.

**Support gatherings.** You can find fellowship and understanding in help bunches where others share comparative difficulties with weight. Check with your PCP, neighborhood emergency clinics or business get-healthy plans for help bunches in your space.

**Weight reduction medicine**

Weight reduction drugs are intended to be utilized alongside diet, exercise and conduct changes, not rather than them. Prior to choosing a drug for you, your primary care physician will think about your well-being history, as well as could be expected incidental effects.

# NORMAL WEIGHT REDUCTION MEDICAL PROCEDURE

**Flexible gastric banding.** In this strategy, an inflatable band isolates the stomach into two pockets. The specialist pulls the band tight, similar to a belt, to make a small channel between the two pockets. The band holds the initial back from extending and is for the most part intended to remain set up for all time.

**Gastric detour a medical procedure.** In gastric detour (Roux-en-Y), the specialist makes a little pocket at the highest point of the stomach. The small digestive system is then stopped a distance underneath the primary stomach and associated with the new pocket. Food and fluid stream straightforwardly from the pocket into this piece of the digestive system, bypassing the greater part of the stomach.

**Gastric sleeve.** In this method, some portion of the stomach is taken out, making a more modest supply for food. It's a less muddled a medical procedure than gastric detour.

Weight reduction accomplishment after medical procedure relies upon your obligation to rolling out deep rooted improvements in your eating and exercise propensities.

# DIFFERENT MEDICINE FOR STOUTNESS

**Hydrogels.** Accessible by remedy, these eatable cases contain little particles that assimilate water and expand in the stomach, to assist you with feeling full. The containers are taken before feasts and are gone through the digestion tracts as stool.

**Vagal nerve bar.** This includes embedding a gadget under the skin of the mid-region that sends discontinuous electrical heartbeats to the stomach vagus nerve, which lets the cerebrum know when the stomach feels vacant or full.

**Gastric suction.** In this method, a cylinder is set through the midsection into the stomach. A piece of the stomach contents are emptied out after every feast.

# WAY OF LIFE AND HOME CURE

Your work to conquer stoutness is bound to find actual success assuming you follow methodologies at home notwithstanding your proper treatment plan. These can include:

**Finding out about your condition.** Training about corpulence can assist you with more deeply studying why you created weight and what can be done. You might feel more engaged to assume command and adhere to your **treatment plan.** Peruse respectable self improvement guides and think about talking regarding them with your primary care physician or specialist.

**Defining reasonable objectives.** At the point when you need to lose a ton of weight, you might put forth objectives that are unreasonable, for example, attempting to lose an excess of excessively quick. Try not to get yourself positioned for disappointment. Put forth day to day or week after week objectives for exercise and weight reduction. Roll out little improvements in your eating routine as opposed to endeavoring extraordinary changes that you're not prone to stay with for the long stretch.

**Adhering to your treatment plan.** Changing a way of life you might have lived with for a long time can be troublesome. Be straightforward with your PCP, advisor or other medical care experts assuming you find your action or eating objectives slipping. You can cooperate to think of novel thoughts or new methodologies.

**Enrolling support.** Get your loved ones ready for your weight reduction objectives. Encircle yourself with individuals who will uphold you and help you, not harm your endeavors. Ensure they comprehend how significant weight reduction is to your well-being. You could likewise need to join a weight reduction support bunch.

**Keeping a record.** Keep a food and movement log. This record can assist you with staying responsible for your eating and exercise propensities. You can find conduct that might be keeping you down and, alternately, what functions admirably for you. You can likewise utilize your log to follow other significant well-being boundaries, for example, circulatory strain and cholesterol levels and generally speaking wellness.

**Elective medication**

Various dietary enhancements that guarantee to assist you with shedding weight rapidly are accessible. The drawn out viability and well-being of these items are frequently sketchy.

## Adapting and support

Converse with your PCP or specialist about further developing your adapting abilities and consider these tips to adapt to corpulence and your weight reduction endeavors:

**Diary.** Write in a diary to communicate torment, outrage, dread or different feelings.

**Associate.** Try not to become segregated. Attempt to partake in standard exercises and get along with family or companions occasionally.

**Join.** Join a care group so you can interface with others confronting comparative difficulties.

**Center.** Remain fixed on your objectives. Defeating weight is a continuous cycle. Remain propelled by remembering your objectives. Advise yourself that you're liable for dealing with your condition and making progress toward your objectives.

**Unwind.** Learn unwinding and stress the executives. Figuring out how to perceive pressure and creating pressure the board and unwinding abilities can assist you with overseeing unfortunate dietary patterns.

Planning for your arrangement

Conversing with your PCP transparently and truly about your weight concerns is perhaps of the smartest option for your well-being. At times, you might be alluded to a corpulence trained professional — in the event that one is accessible in your space. You may likewise be alluded to a social instructor or dietitian.

# CONCLUSIONS: WHAT YOU CAN DO

Being a functioning member in your consideration is significant. One method for doing this is by getting ready for your arrangement. Contemplate your requirements and objectives for treatment. Likewise, record a rundown of inquiries to pose. These inquiries might include:

What eating or movement propensities are reasonable adding to my well-being concerns and weight gain?

What might I at any point do about the difficulties I look in dealing with my weight?

Do I have other medical conditions that are brought about by corpulence?

Would it be a good idea for me to see a dietitian?

Would it be a good idea for me to see a conduct guide with skill in weight the executives?

What are the treatment choices for heftiness and my other medical issues?

Is weight reduction intercession a possibility for me?

Make certain to tell your primary care physician about any ailments you have and about any prescriptions, nutrients or enhancements that you take.

What's in store from your primary care physician

During your arrangement, your primary care physician is probably going to pose you various inquiries about your weight, eating, action, mind-set and considerations, and any side effects you could have. You might be posed such inquiries as:

What amount did you show up secondary school?

What life altering situations might have been related with weight gain?

What and what amount do you eat in a common day?

How much movement do you get in a commonplace day?

During what times of your life did you put on weight?

What are the elements that you trust influence your weight?

How is your day to day routine impacted by your weight?

What diets or medicines have you attempted to get more fit?

What are your weight reduction objectives?

Might it be said that you are prepared to make changes in your way of life to get more fit?

What might keep you from getting thinner?

What you can do meanwhile

On the off chance that have opportunity and willpower before your booked arrangement, you can help get ready for the arrangement by saving an eating regimen journal for a very long time preceding the arrangement and by recording the number of steps you require in a day by utilizing a stage counter (pedometer).

You can likewise start to go with decisions that will assist you with beginning to shed pounds, including:

Rolling out sound improvements in your eating regimen. Incorporate more natural products, vegetables and entire grains in your eating regimen. Start to decrease segment sizes.

**Expanding your movement level.** Attempt to often get up and move around your home more. Begin bit by bit on the off chance that you're not looking great or aren't accustomed to working out. Indeed, even a 10-minute day to day walk can help. In the event that you have any medical issue or are over a specific age — more than 40 for men and north of 50 for ladies — hold on until you've conversed with your primary care physician before you start another activity program.

www.ingramcontent.com/pod-product-compliance
Lightning Source LLC
LaVergne TN
LVHW020542160826
845677LV00015B/4158
* 9 7 9 8 8 4 6 1 5 4 3 0 8 *